DEDICATION

With appreciation for the community of mothers and
grandmothers who have made my own journey possible.
With hope to aid other travelers on their journeys…

CONTENTS

ACKNOWLEDGMENTS

This booklet, and all of my breastfeeding support work, was made possible by Connie Culley who first gave me a ride, and then gave me her insight, mentorship, friendship, and support. Hana Askren has been the enthusiastic and skilled editor I needed to keep this project moving forward. Hilary Flower wrote the original book on Tandem Nursing that got me started on this path. The community of Tandem Nursing discussion groups on Facebook helped me along on my own journey, and showed me the need for more maps and tools to further guide the way. My mother showed me, by living it fully, the core principle of so much of breastfeeding and parenting – *Trust Your Instincts*. My father, through his life's work helping both children and adults, taught me to respect the significance of the emotional life of children of all ages. My family has supported and put up with my absorption in this project, and my husband Ben has been an important sounding board. Of course, all the errors contained within are mine alone.

i

INTRODUCTION

When I started my own tandem nursing journey, I was lucky enough to be supported by an experienced group of mothers and grandmothers through La Leche League. Still, I often looked for and sought more support, joining several tandem nursing groups on-line, and, as my experience and confidence grew, attempting to offer support to others through these groups as well. I saw many posts from mothers seeking more resources; since there seemed to be a need for more written resources, I decided to write this guide.

I hope that this Pocket Guide *to Tandem Nursing is a useful and concise introduction for families considering tandem nursing. For further information, I hope you will seek out your local Breastfeeding Peer Support Group and other forms of community support.*

While finalizing this Pocket Guide, *I heard the welcome news* that the classic book Adventures in Tandem Nursing *was being updated and will be back in print and available again before too long. If you are seeking further written resources, I recommend it for the most comprehensive catalog of the experiences of scores of families, in depth information on tandem related topics, clear explanations of some of the science behind lactation, and the definitive summary of available research.*

I am excited to be able to finally share this Pocket Guide. *Breastfeeding a baby, and Tandem Nursing, are such remarkable experiences, and such an amazing way of nurturing our children. I hope this* Pocket Guide *can help you to get started on your unique journey, and that every family can go forward finding all the resources they need to make informed breastfeeding choices!*

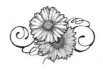

1 WHY TANDEM NURSE?

Tandem nursing is breastfeeding more than one child during the same time period. It can be simultaneous, with a child latched to each breast at the same time, or in succession, at different points during the day. The children may be different ages, or they may be twins / multiples of the same age.

Why do families choose to tandem nurse? The reasons are as many and varied as families themselves. Some common reasons include:

- ❖ Providing to the older child the continued health benefits of perhaps the most nutritious food on earth.

- ❖ Maintaining the emotional bond of breastfeeding.

- ❖ Easing the toddler's transition from youngest to elder.

❖ Keeping the magical comfort tool of breastfeeding in the parenting toolbox, always at hand to ease the inevitable (both physical and emotional) bumps and bruises of toddler life.

❖ Reinforcing and supporting the bond between siblings.

❖ In the case of twins / multiples, simply the desire to provide babies with their optimal food.

2 NURSING CHALLENGES

Tandem nursing, like nursing a single child, comes with plenty of challenges. Breastfeeding is the most "natural" thing in the world, and yet it does not always "come naturally". Many first time parents have never actually seen a baby breastfeed. And most have never even imagined, let alone seen, two children nursing at the same time.

Breastfeeding has a learned, as well as an instinctual component. But an abundance of cultural knowledge that in the past would have been passed down through extended families and close knit, family centered communities, is no longer accessible to many parents in the modern world. To learn the basics, and overcome the hurdles, parents need *all* the support and accurate information that they can get, from other parents, from trained Peer Support Counselors, from lactation professionals, from online discussion groups and websites, and from written materials.

Can I nurse during pregnancy? Is it safe? How do I manage the competing needs of newborn and older sibling? How do I fit two babies on the breast? And what about bedtimes? All of these concrete questions need concrete answers.

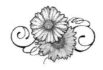

3 HOW DID I GET HERE?

Many families begin their nursing journeys without imagining that they will be nursing past the first few months, let alone the first year. And yet, as our babies grow, we see that they are continuing to benefit both physically and emotionally from breastfeeding. The American Academy of Pediatrics (AAP) recommends breastfeeding to "one year or longer as mutually desired by mother and infant...."[1] The World Health Organization (WHO) raises this to a recommendation of "...up to two years of age or beyond."[2]

Readiness for full weaning, like so many other developmental milestones, comes at different points for different parent / child groupings. Parents who choose to follow "child-led weaning", responding to a child's cues as they have from the start of the

[1] American Academy of Pediatrics, Section on Breastfeeding. Policy statement: breastfeeding and the use of human milk. Pediatrics. 2012;129[3]:e827–e841

[2] World Health Organization: Global Strategy on Infant and Child Feeding,2002

nursing relationship, find that even different children within the same family will choose to wean on vastly different schedules. So many factors can play a role, from temperament, to physical health, to food sensitivity, to emotional strains. And of course, all of these factors come to bear on adults as well, and will affect your willingness and ability to continue nursing your child.

For those families that have chosen (and been able) to continue nursing past infancy, or when a pregnancy occurs very early in a new baby's life, whether to tandem nurse suddenly becomes an immediate decision.

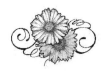

4 BREASTFEEDING AND PREGNANCY

Breastfeeding during pregnancy comes with its own set of challenges-- from concerns about safety and milk production, to nipple soreness, and aversions. But it also brings some special joys and advantages. Even the most energetic toddler is often happy to lie down and nurse when given the opportunity. Getting that quiet time with your child can make it a lot easier to get off your feet, which is a big help when you are pregnant with a little one in tow. And the cozy time with your child is particularly precious to both of you as you prepare for a new baby and weather the ups and downs of pregnancy.

Safety

For many years, healthcare professionals were concerned that the effects of breastfeeding on hormones during pregnancy could contribute to premature labor. Breastfeeding stimulates oxytocin release, and oxytocin is associated with uterine contractions. But current research on *healthy, low risk* pregnancies has *not* found any association between breastfeeding and premature labor, low birth weight, preeclampsia, or any other pregnancy complications.[3]

Current medical understanding suggests that the uterus does not develop the oxytocin receptors that could be stimulated by oxytocin release until very late in pregnancy, and so breastfeeding alone would not stimulate premature labor.[4]

Many families consider the guideline of "pelvic rest" (i.e. medical advice to avoid sex) when evaluating the risk that breastfeeding could pose to a given pregnancy. Sexual climax releases higher levels of oxytocin than breastfeeding does, and stimulates uterine contractions as well. In a pregnancy in which pelvic rest is prescribed, avoiding breastfeeding would seem to be a logical precaution to be considered. If pelvic rest is *not* prescribed, breastfeeding would seem to be a lesser risk.

Of course, every individual medical situation needs to be considered on its own individual merits, and with the advice of a health care practitioner who is aware of the full health history involved. In general, most health care practitioners now advise that breastfeeding is safe during healthy pregnancies, as stated in American Academy of Family Physicians (AAFP) recommendations, "...Breastfeeding during a subsequent

---

[3] Madarshahian, Hassanabadi M, *J Nurs Res*. 2012 Mar;20(1):74-80; Ishii H, *J Obstet Gynaecol Res*. 2009 Oct;35(5):864-8, for additional resources see Flower, Hilary. "Breastfeeding During Pregnancy and Tandem Nursing: Is it Safe? Recent Research." *Breastfeeding Today* April 2016.

[4] Kimura T. et al, Expression of Oxytocin Receptor in Human Pregnant Myometrium, *Endocrinology* 1996; 137: 780-785

pregnancy is not unusual. If the pregnancy is normal and the mother is healthy, breastfeeding during pregnancy is the woman's personal decision. If the child is younger than two years, the child is at increased risk of illness if weaned."[5]

Whether or not breastfeeding during pregnancy is the right choice for you is a highly individual and personal decision that each family must make for themselves, ideally with the input of a knowledgeable health care professional. No choice is without disadvantages. Ending breastfeeding also carries its own drawbacks for both child and parent, as well as emotional implications. All these aspects must be weighed against each other in any decision, and only the family involved has the full picture needed to strike this balance.

Unfortunately, there is a very normal background risk of pregnancy loss that exists irrespective of breastfeeding. About 1 in 3 of all pregnancies do end in miscarriages during the first few months. So it is important for every breastfeeding family to feel confident in their breastfeeding decision, and to be at peace, regardless of how the pregnancy progresses, that they have made the best decision for their own unique situation.

In cases where a miscarriage does occur, it's important not to second guess a decision to continue breastfeeding. There's usually no reason to think breastfeeding caused the loss, and second guessing only adds pain to an already difficult situation. And, if weaning is undertaken before mother and child are fully ready, and then a pregnancy is lost, it can add to the difficulty of the loss.

To make the best decision, families need access to accurate

---

[5] AAFP Position Statement on Breastfeeding. 2008.

information. And then, as with many aspects of parenting, we need to *trust our instincts*, and feel confident and that we have come to a decision that feels right to us, not based on outside influences in either direction.

Milk Supply

As a pregnancy progresses, most mothers experience a reduced supply of milk. This may be most apparent to mothers who pump regularly, but mothers who feed exclusively at the breast may notice their toddlers nursing more often and switching sides more frequently, or becoming frustrated by slower flow. As with so many things in pregnancy and birth, there is a great deal of individual variation.

According to one study, about 70% of pregnant breast feeders notice a significant decline in milk supply by the middle of their pregnancies, when pregnancy hormones displace milk removal as the leading determinant of supply. But another 30% do not experience a significant reduction in supply and are able to continue breastfeeding unabated.[6]

As supply decreases, the flavor of the milk changes. Some little ones may choose to stop nursing at this point because they dislike the flavor. (Some of these same will still happily resume again, if given the option, after the new baby arrives and a flush of new milk comes in.) But many nurslings will continue nursing with relish, regardless of what is, or is not, coming out of the

---

[6] Moscone S, Moore M., Breastfeeding During Pregnancy. *J Hum Lact.* 1993; 9(2):83-88.

nipple.

Towards the middle of a pregnancy (though there is a variety in timing, as well), milk changes over to colostrum in preparation for the new baby. Again some little ones will balk at the change, while others are unfazed.

If your nursling is under the age of one year, or an older child who has not taken to solids yet, you will want to stay in touch with your pediatrician and keep a close eye on weight and nutrition to ensure that nurslings get what they need while milk supply potentially dwindles. In general, children under one year still need to receive the bulk of their nutrition from breastmilk or an artificial breastmilk substitute, i.e. "formula". It can be necessary to supplement these young ones, whether with donor breast milk if a safe source is available, or with commercial formula. (Where available, donor human milk is generally the preferred choice for supplementing.[7])

Older children over one year may be able to simply increase their intake of nutritious solid foods to meet basic nutritional needs, if breastmilk supply dwindles.

If you have been working and pumping you may find that you are suddenly unable to pump much. Many pumping parents feel ready to wean from the pump around the time their child turns a year old in any case, but you can continue to offer the breast to your child when you are together, even if you are no longer pumping at work. If your child is under the age of one, or not yet eating many solid foods, then you should talk with your pediatrician about choosing an appropriate breastmilk

---

[7] Wambach K, Riordan J, Breastfeeding and Human Lactation 5th ed 2016; 10:391

substitute. Otherwise, with older children who are eating solids well, nutritious solid foods can take up the slack.

Even when a nursling is getting added supplement or solid food, whatever milk they are able to get from *you* is giving them valuable immune and digestive support and nutrition, not to mention emotional comfort. So it can still be very worthwhile to continue nursing as long as parent and child continue to desire it.

Soreness & Aversions

Nipple soreness and nursing aversions are associated with the special cocktail of hormones that support pregnancy. They will often come and go or ebb and flow over the course of a pregnancy. There is a great variety in the severity with which mothers experience these symptoms, from minor annoyance, to excruciating, to barely resistible urges to push away and flee.

What can we make of these sensations? If you are pregnant and nursing and have not experienced them, don't worry! It may be that you never will! If you are however, finding yourself somewhere on this spectrum, it may help, first off, to realize that you are not alone! This is a fairly common experience, and it is driven by your hormones and has no bearing on your dedication to breastfeeding, or your love for your nursling. There are several things you can try to make it better, or at least more bearable.

A range of responses have been helpful to other breastfeeding parents in this situation:

Address Latch

Toddlers and older babies are famous for gymnastic feats while nursing. They are nursing pros, and tend to get careless about how they latch as well as distracted by other thoughts and activities while in the midst of nursing. They will attempt to nurse from all sorts of awkward positions. They are also often verbal enough to understand directions about opening their mouths wide and sticking out their tongues, and are able to become partners in an effort to improve the nursing relationship. A sloppy latch that didn't cause pain before pregnancy can be the last straw after pregnancy hormones kick in!

Nursing in a quiet space, where both of you can focus all of your attention on the nursing and the latch, and making it clear to your nursling what positions feel good and which don't, can sometimes make a big difference in your comfort.

Supporting your breast with your own hand while nursing can both improve the depth of the latch, and create more of a feeling of control which many mothers find can help combat nursing aversions.

Although a spirited little one may resist efforts to restrain squirming, "twiddling" with the other nipple, and other behaviors which can suddenly become intolerable, the child who is very attached to nursing may surprise you with a willingness to cooperate once you make it clear that this is the only path to the precious treat of continued nursing.

Taking Care

Making space for personal or alone time, or for favorite activities that may have slipped off your priority list due to the demands of parenthood, can be an important, even essential, investment that pays dividends for everyone in the family. Doing some of the things that help you to unwind and "refill your cup" can raise your threshold for irritation, and bring out infinitely more energy and creativity to address all the varied challenges that arise in every parenting day, breastfeeding related or otherwise. And of course, seemingly simple things like making sure you are drinking enough water and eating well are important too, as are getting naps if you are short on sleep.

Visualization

Visualization can be a valuable tool in mitigating aversions. One way to go about this: Think about the things that you value most about breastfeeding. Then picture them in action as you are nursing. Imagine you can see the glowing love flowing out of you towards your child as she slowly fills to the brim with colorful warmth and light. Or picture superhero immunities streaming through your body and breasts and out into your nursling. Experiment with different pictures until you find something that moves (and distracts!) you.

Limits

In conjunction with all of the above, many experiencing aversions choose to limit a child's time at the breast. Strategies for doing this can be tailored to your child's temperament and level of development and understanding, and be consistent with any parenting style you already practice in other areas. Some creative tools that many families have found helpful:

❖ Choose (or let child choose) a song, and nurse for the duration of the song only.

❖ Ask your child to choose a number. Nurse for as long as it takes you to count to that number. Depending on your mood, and how high the number, you can count fast or slow - kids rarely seem to notice the difference, and you can stay in control of the duration this way, while giving your child a sense of control and predictability as well.

❖ Give your older child a certain number of markers for the day (checkers, poker chips, bottle caps, whatever seems fun that you have on hand), which can be redeemed for nursing sessions during the course of the day.

❖ Brainstorm about what variety of needs your child is expressing and meeting through nursing. Then look for alternatives that meet some of these same needs, and provide these alternatives, if possible *before* the child even asks to nurse. For example, offer frequent chewy snacks and camelback style water bottles for both oral stimulation as well as calories and hydration. If you think your child may be seeking sensory stimulation, make a point of lots of hugs and cuddles, plus rough housing if fun for extra physical contact. Other family members can help with this too.

Don't Sit Down

Well, maybe not the best plan when pregnant! But do try to be out and about at playgroups, library story hours, running errands, taking walks, etc., to keep your child distracted from nursing and interested in the outside world.

Just Say No

Tell your child it doesn't feel good to nurse right now, and be clear about when, or how often, your child will be able to nurse again. Perhaps you want to nurse at bedtimes and naptimes only, or only in a certain location. With verbal children, make it clear that this is about how your body feels. Try not to blame the baby, or the nursing child. Some parents put bandaids on their breasts and explain that they have "ouchies", or whatever term the child is familiar with from their own experience of minor cuts and bruises, to indicate the times when nursing is not available.

Night Weaning

Many families choose to night wean their older baby before or during pregnancy. It's important to note, however, that as one sleep deprived mama put it, "Public Service Announcement: Night Weaning does not always equal more sleep!" Breastfeeding is a highly effective sleep inducer, and removing that tool from the parenting tool box does sometimes mean just as many night wakings, but more time and effort spent getting a child back to sleep. Some kids will stop waking immediately, others after a few tough nights, but still others not for quite some time. Temperament and developmental readiness for sleeping through the night vary a great deal among little ones.

When they are ready, or nearly so, a small nudge, and help from a non-nursing partner or other supportive adult to comfort them during the night may be enough to painlessly night wean little ones. But if they are not ready, it can be quite an ordeal for all involved. Sometimes the only way to know how it will go is to give it a try, but you may want to be prepared to change plans if you feel that the process is taking too great a toll.

Although more sleep isn't necessarily a result that you can count on, if you are feeling a need to reduce breastfeeding, and especially if you have a partner or supportive adult present who is able to help with nighttime parenting, night weaning can be a helpful strategy. Many families find that it eases the process to prepare the child in advance with discussion about what to expect, and spend time reading children's books together about night weaning, such as *Nursies When the Sun Shines* by Katherine Havener (Elea Press; 2013). Some families even create their own book, with photos from their own family pasted into the pages.

Complete Weaning

Some families find that breastfeeding during pregnancy is just not working for them. Aversions may be too intense, or other complications may arise and you will need to take the lead in weaning. Or your little one may take the lead, disliking the new flavor of milk or the lack of milk. Those little ones who wean during pregnancy may completely lose interest, or may forget how to latch if they are given the chance to try in the future. On the other hand, some will be happy to pick up right where they left off after the new baby arrives, if you wish to offer them the option.

If you do choose to wean, and wish your child to remain weaned, there is much you can do to provide other types of closeness, and to remind your little one of all the great activities and foods that an older baby or toddler can partake in, but the new baby cannot.

Nursing is a relationship and it has to work for both parties. Many families find that pregnancy is a natural time for weaning. You are always free to make the choice to end nursing, and continuing to nurse if you feel resentment about it can be counterproductive for all involved. Some breastfeeding parents find that once they "give themselves permission" to wean, they begin to feel more positively about nursing, and choose to continue. Others find that weaning is the best choice for their unique combination of circumstances and temperaments. Every family will have to find their own balance for their own unique situation.

5 PREPARING FOR A NEW NURSLING

As your little one's awareness of the

pregnancy grows, you have an opportunity to shape perceptions and lay some groundwork for the future sibling relationship. The words you use to describe the impending upheaval can influence how your older nursling processes it. For this reason many families make an effort to assign credit to the baby and avoid blame.

When pregnancy is disruptive for your little one, look for a way to put it into context as part of your child growing, or of parents having their own needs, rather than being a direct result of the baby. When you are tired, try, "I need to rest, will you come and snuggle with me?" rather than, "Being pregnant makes me tired." When nursing your little one is uncomfortable, "I am sore right now, I need to take a break," rather than, "Being pregnant makes me sore, I need to take a break." When milk changes taste or dwindles, "You are a big kid now, and my body knows you don't need so much milk. When the new baby comes, she will make lots of milk for both of you to share." Rather than "My body needs to take care of the baby now, instead of making milk for you."

For both parents and children, it can be helpful to frame each thought in the context of abundance, "There are more children and the pie gets bigger!", rather than scarcity, "There are more children splitting the same sized pie." At least in the case of milk supply, this is tangibly true.

When you have one little one fully occupying all of your available time and attention, it can be hard to imagine how you will care for, and love, a second on top of all that. It is true that more children add complexity, but many families find that each new being adds so much more, and somehow makes space for themselves. As one grandmother explained to her adult daughter expecting number two, "The first one opens up your heart, and the rest fall right in."

6 THE BABY ARRIVES

Your tender newborn is finally here, resting in your arms. The time has come for your older baby and newborn to meet. There are a few things you may wish to take into consideration to help things get off on the right foot.

Your Own Feelings

Many parents report that their older baby, who seemed so small and gentle and vulnerable the day before the new birth, now suddenly appears more like a huge, blundering, awkward elephant. The magic of perspective can change things in an instant. And the rush of birth hormones can create a tremendous protective instinct towards the new baby that alters the picture.

Your Child's Feelings

Imagine you have been the center of your family's world for as long as you can remember. Then, sometime recently, there began to be lots of commotion and distraction in your house. People seemed excited. If you are old enough to be verbal, you've been asked countless, enthusiastic questions about your "new brother or sister" by well meaning adults. Perhaps you're curious about what this is really all about, or just impatient with all the talk and distracted focus. It seems to go on forever but not lead to anything you can see, besides less milk flow when you nurse, and a protruding belly that gets in the way sometimes. Why all the upheaval? Things were quite nice the way they were before, with you squarely in the center.

To make matters worse, mom suddenly goes into labor and withdraws completely, either physically disappearing from your view, or, even if you are present for any of the process, withdrawing into the tunnel vision of labor.

To dramatize the potential tenderness of an older sibling's perspective, Faber and Mazlish in their book *Siblings Without Rivalry* (W. W. Nortan & Co.; 2012) use this example: How would you feel if you had a Significant Other who announced one day, "I love having you as a my husband / wife / partner so much, I've decided to add another one!"?

Your Newborn's Feelings

Newborns need and expect constant warmth, touch, and frequent doses of breast milk, whenever they reach out. They are not conscious of much else, at first.

Striking A Balance

How do tandem families balance these disparate views?

Keep your older baby's perspective in mind. If another adult besides you can be holding the newborn for the first meeting, your older baby can have your full attention, and perhaps even nurse alone, finding reassurance that her place in the world is still secure.

Almost inevitably the moment will arise when older baby and newborn want to nurse at the same time. Think in advance about how you might want to handle this. Some families feel it is important to teach older children to wait. Others may choose to nurse both children simultaneously, one on each breast, or even to give the older nursling some opportunities to be "first". You are the best judge of your child's temperament and development. How much can she handle? How does it feel to *you*?

Keep in mind that a newborn, unlike an older child, has no sense of "fairness", and no fear of being displaced. A newborn is not drawing conclusions from each interaction. Many older children will be watching closely, and whatever choices you make will communicate something to your older nursling. On the other hand, a newborn *does* need to nurse often, and *you* do need to be comfortable and to rest and recover from birth.

Which choices best balance all of these needs will be unique for each family and yet another occasion where you will do best by following your own instincts, unclouded by the potential judgments of others.

Some families find that their child is ready and able to wait for the newborn to nurse, and that even if this leads to some frustration, it proves to be a valuable lesson and works best for parents and children. On the other hand, some families discover that pushing their little one to wait during this vulnerable time creates jealousy and makes nursing into a battle that only brings extra difficulty for all.

If you and baby are comfortable nursing two together at the same time, one on each breast, this can be a simple solution. Sometimes a middle ground helps as well, for example making a point to the older child that the newborn has to be allowed to latch on first and given a certain predictable amount of time on the breast alone, and then the older sibling will be allowed to join in on the other breast. It often takes two adult hands to help a newborn latch and stay on the breast securely, whilst an older baby can get on and stay on unassisted. Letting the newborn latch first leaves two hands free for the newborn.

Often it takes families some time to find the right balance in their new circumstances. The process can work most smoothly where there is openness to different possibilities, communication amongst the adults as everyone's emotions and circumstances evolve, and perhaps most important of all, a healthy sense of humor!

Above all, if it's not working, change something! Although consistency of approach can be reassuring to little ones, sticking with something that isn't working for anyone is rarely helpful. Consistency can be more about style, approach, and values. How your family applies those to the specifics of each new and always evolving situation may require flexibility in order to find the most workable approach.

The early days of nursing two are another opportunity to give your older child a positive framework for the budding sibling relationship. Look for opportunities to credit the baby for all things good. And when things are difficult for the older sibling, try looking for a broader explanation, and avoid "blaming" the newborn baby.

During your pregnancy your milk supply may have dwindled, and the taste and composition will have changed from mature milk for the toddler, to colostrum for the baby. Just a few days after the new baby arrives, there is a flush of milk which delights most older nurslings. It can be helpful to loudly credit the baby for its role in "making" this great milk, and "sharing" it with an older sibling.

7 WILL OLDER BABY STEAL NEWBORN'S MILK?

Many families are understandably concerned that the milk babies need will be "used up" by an older nursling. Human milk has the almost magical property of becoming more abundant the more it is removed. Milk will not be "used up", but it is still very important to nurse the newborn baby often. Babies need to nurse frequently, and latch and transfer milk effectively, in order to get the milk they need. When babies remove milk effectively, and spend plenty of time at the breast, most nursing parents make plenty for two, just as they would for twins (or, for that matter triplets) of the same age.

All newborns, whether singleton or tandem nurslings, need to be observed to ensure that they are swallowing at the breast, producing the appropriate number of wet and dirty diapers for their age, and, most importantly, gaining weight at an appropriate rate. If they are doing these things, they are getting enough milk.

If healthy full term infants are held skin to skin, and their families are responding to their cues, they will nurse frequently. If older nurslings are interfering with this process, or if you are feeling overwhelmed by the older nursling's demands, then you will need to set more limits on your older nursling. If babies are given pacifiers, or swaddled and placed in cribs, all of which may discourage feeding or mask feeding cues, then extra attention will need to be applied to ensure that babies are given enough opportunities to nurse. ***But scarcity of milk does not in itself need to be a concern for tandem feeders!***

8 CHOOSING SIDES

Whether or not to assign a side to each child is really a matter of preference. Different families do this differently. Some child pairs arrive at a division without adult intervention, and some parents will find it easiest to just stick with whatever their kids have arrived at. Some parents feel most comfortable assigning sides. We do know that one breast alone can provide enough to sustain a baby.

Assigned sides can lead to uneven breast sizes in the short term, but most parents report that sizes even out again after weaning. Many who do not assign sides or who are nursing only one child still report that one side produces significantly more than another, and remains a different size as long as lactation continues.

Some chiropractors have suggested that when babies switch sides it aids in neurological and muscular development. Changing positions even when nursing on only one side may help to create some of the same benefits.

The process of changing sides, or negotiating sides, can be a source of conflict for some nursing pairs, although it can also be an opportunity for positive associations and learning. Very young babies often don't care which side they are on, and in this case, giving the older nursling the option to choose a side at each nursing session, and even going through the motions of thanking the preverbal younger for granting the wish, can be very reassuring to the older nursling. If you do mix sides, starting this ritual early, before a younger baby cares at all, can create a positive template to follow as the siblings age. Navigating this potential conflict as siblings grow, with your presence and support, can give siblings tools to use in the inevitable push and pull of family (and all) life that will follow.

Some parents are concerned that when children switch sides, they may receive the "wrong" fat content, or "kind" of milk. In fact, your body only produces one type of milk, and as long as your children are nursing frequently, the fat will not separate out of the milk to such a significant degree. When babies are put on a feeding schedule with long gaps between feedings, the fat will start to settle and stick to the milk ducts, and the early milk that comes out in a feeding will have significantly less fat diluted in it, then as the feeding continues, the fat will gradually mix back in. Frequent feeding on cue will avoid this issue in most cases, and any minor differences in fat content that ensue will even themselves out over the course of a day of frequent nursing.

When you go through pregnancy, your hormones take control of your milk production, and your milk resets to colostrum which provides the perfect nutritional content for your newborn. This will still be nutritious for your older nursling. But whichever breast your children are on, your younger and older children will both be receiving milk that is tailored for the youngest. There is still some responsiveness to the older nursling though-- scientists have theorized that pathogens present in the saliva of *either* nursling will stimulate production of appropriate antibodies in the breastfeeding parent's immune system, which will then be passed back through the milk to support the immune systems of all nurslings!

What about when one child is sick? Germs do have a way of traveling around families, and by the time either child shows symptoms of an illness, it generally means that both have already been exposed. While some parents may try to separate the nurslings at this point and designate sides and/or attempt a thorough cleaning regimen between nursing each child, many others feel their time is better spent nursing each as often as possible to share the immune supporting antibodies in their milk.

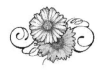

9 TODDLER TURMOIL

Many older babies and toddlers exhibit some stressed behaviors in the first few months after the birth of a new sibling. Children who are tandem nursing are no exception, and different children will exhibit stresses in different ways. They often have shorter fuses, more frequent tantrums, more obstinate moments, less self control, toilet training regression, or more bouts of aggressive hitting or biting than they did before the new baby arrived. Older babies who have the opportunity often increase their nursing frequency dramatically, and some even begin cutting back on or refusing solid food in favor of nursing.

This rocky period can be tough to handle for parents trying to find a new equilibrium while caring for an expanded family and meeting the needs of a newborn. Sometimes it helps just to know how common it is -- so many other families have experienced the same thing!

In the very early days with a newborn, when friends or family offer to help, often the most helpful thing of all that they can do can be playing with your older baby, showering her with attention, or if possible taking him on excursions out of the house so that you can focus on nursing your newborn.

When you are ready to be more active yourself, learning to nurse your youngest baby in a baby carrier can leave your hands and attention free for your older child, while you are still frequently nursing your littlest. This is especially helpful if you have one of those toddlers who are reminded that they want to nurse every time they see the baby nurse. Often these same toddlers will not notice when the baby in the carrier is nursing, especially when you are out in the world together with plenty of distractions for toddler to focus on.

Another strategy many families use for keeping an older baby busy while the youngest nurses (if you don't want to nurse them alongside the baby every time) is to designate a special basket of toys or favorite activities for the elder to use only while the baby nurses.

All the various strategies for limiting nursing that were discussed in the pregnancy nursing section earlier can be helpful to consider during the postpartum phase as well.

Another approach that often helps to calm stressed older siblings is to carve out a predictable, daily time when you can give the bigger sibling your undivided, one-on-one attention. No phone, texts, etc., just a one-on-one time, talking, reading, or playing, or even doing a chore together with no distractions (as long as it is one in which your child can fully participate, and it does not take your attention away from your child). Often while your youngest naps is the most practical time to do this. Even a short time period can be very helpful.

Although it can be hard to carve out the time, many parents find that doing so pays dividends in improved behavior throughout the day that make it a worthwhile time investment. In fact many parents report that this can be a helpful parenting strategy to return to long after weaning -- focused, one-on-one time can be a balm in many different situations, ages, and stages.

10 POSITIONS... LOGISTICS...

How can you fit two children on your breasts at the same time? The answers to this question are many and various-- as many ways as there are nursing trios! To start out with a newborn and an older baby, it is often helpful to begin in a reclined, "laid back" position. This is a great way to start with a newborn alone, using gravity as an ally to help baby get a deep latch, and harnessing baby's natural instinct to squirm up your chest, find your breast, and latch on. Breastfeeding helpers remind us that our breasts are circles of 360 degrees, and nurslings can latch from any direction that is comfortable. So if, for example, you have had a C-section birth and need to avoid pressure on an incision site, a nursling can lie over your shoulder and latch from above.

Once baby is comfortably latched, older nurslings can be very flexible. They can stand, kneel, perch on your knee, drape over your shoulder, lie by your side -- they will find a way. To see pictures and glean ideas about the variety of ways that tandem families go about arranging themselves, it can be very helpful to join one of the tandem nursing Facebook discussion groups such as "La Leche League - Tandem Nursing" where families post photos and swap ideas.

Above all, make sure that you, the breastfeeding parent, are comfortable. Add pillows to support your back, neck, or arms. Avoid leaning over a nursling -- as the saying goes: "Bring the baby to the breast, not the breast to the baby". Unlatch whenever you have nipple pain by placing your finger in the corner of your baby's mouth to break the suction. Then try again to get a deeper latch by holding your nursling closer to your body and making sure they are opening WIDE and getting a full mouthful of breast, not just nipple. Helping them to approach the breast from below, nose lined up with your nipple to start, can encourage a wider gape and fuller mouthful.

Whether you are nursing single or tandem, if your newborn's latch is not working, ask for help right away! Contact your local La Leche League, or Breastfeeding USA, or call an IBCLC. If you are in a hospital after a birth, ask to see the hospital lactation specialist, not just the postpartum nurse who may have little or no training in breastfeeding help beyond sometimes limited personal experience.

If you have any significant pain, regardless of how latch "looks" on the outside, it is a sign that the latch is not functioning properly -- this can damage your breast, and reduce the amount of milk flowing to your baby.

Breastfeeding parents have extraordinary strength and determination when they are working to meet the needs of their babies. But putting up with pain without getting help to address it is ignoring an important signal from your body, and can make the situation worse for both you and your baby. Don't hesitate to ask for the help you *and* your baby need! And seek out skilled helpers who can provide it.

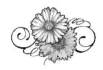

11 BEDTIME

How do you put two nursing children to bed? Well, as one tandem mama put it, "How on earth do you put a non-nursing child to bed?" Caring for two young children at the same time can be trying under most circumstances. Many parents find that nursing is actually a wonderful, soporific tool that can put children to sleep more quickly than most. But bedtimes are often a juggle regardless of your tool box. If you are comfortable nursing simultaneously, you may find that lying down reclined with a few pillows behind you for support and a little one on each side is a very quick way to put all three of you to sleep, especially in the early weeks after birth. If you want your nurslings to sleep on separate surfaces during the night, you may also find that one or both will be heavily enough asleep after several minutes that you can shift their positions and move them onto separate surfaces.

If you have a partner or other support person available at bedtime who can help, you may want to nurse one child to sleep first while your partner is with the other, and then switch. If that is not an option, you may be able to find a special quiet activity that your toddler is able to undertake independently while you nurse the baby to sleep -- something special that is taken out only at bedtimes. And whatever strategy works at one stage may need to change as your children grow or your own needs and schedule changes.

Of course, if you choose to bed share, it's important to keep in mind the "Safe Sleep 7" Guidelines.

Safe bed sharing requires:

A parent who is:

1. A non-smoker

2. Sober (No alcohol, no sleep inducing medications.)

3. Breastfeeding

A baby who is:

4. Healthy

5. On his back

6. Lightly dressed and un-swaddled

And they must share:

7. a safe surface (No super soft mattress, no extra pillows, no toys, no heavy covers. Clear of strings and cords. Pack the cracks: use rolled towels or baby blankets.)

For more details on safe bed sharing, see the book *Sweet Sleep* by Wiessinger et al. (Ballentine Books; 2014)

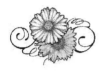

12 BACK TO WORK

If you are returning to work, or other regular separation from your baby, you may wonder if allowing your older nursling to continue nursing will create added complication in what is already a challenging juggle of responsibilities. The good news is that many of the benefits of tandem nursing can actually be of extra help to working and breastfeeding parents.

Many pumping parents choose to stop pumping at work when their children have reached one year old or so, and the child's intake of table foods has become the main source of their nutrition. After the age of one, it is generally not necessary to supplement with formula, even when breastmilk is unavailable for stretches of the day. Any amount of breastmilk is still extremely beneficial for the immunities and nutrition it provides, prompting major health organizations such as the World Health Organization (WHO) to recommend continued nursing through age two and beyond. But this benefit can be achieved by simply nursing an older child when you are together, without the need to pump during separations. So, for most tandem nursing pumping parents, your pumping output will be primarily designated for your younger baby.

If you are pumping at work to provide milk for your younger nursling, you may find that you are able to pump out more milk, more quickly, due to the extra stimulation that your older nursling provides by breastfeeding when you are together. Assuming that you are only pumping for your younger child while you are separated, you now have more supply available to draw from for the younger.

If you have found comfortable ways to breastfeed your two nurslings simultaneously, you may find that nursing together when you are reunited is a great way to reconnect calmly with both, right away.

Pumping is a big commitment, and coordinating multiple child care arrangements and the needs of additional children is always going to be a challenge, however you are feeding your little ones. If you are finding tandem nursing stressful, it may be harder to push through some of these obstacles while also juggling separations and work responsibilities. You may need to consider setting more limits, or change your tandem plan all together. But if you are able to find your groove with tandem nursing, and it is going smoothly, tandem nursing can be a tool that actually simplifies your busy days.

13 PUTTING IT ALL TOGETHER

Pregnant nursing and Tandem nursing

bring challenges. While they are not for everyone, current research suggests that they are a safe path for those with healthy, low risk pregnancies. Countless tandem families have found them to be a rewarding way to nurture a growing family. For those able to find support and strength to navigate soreness, aversions, and other challenges along the way, tandem nursing is a wonderful option to have.

It is, of course, hard to know in advance what needs will emerge in our children and ourselves, and what circumstances will ask of us. If we can take one step at a time, responding to the moment we are in, and balancing the needs of the whole family, we can find the path that works best for us-- whether that be a child or parent led weaning, or a brief or extended tandem nursing relationship.

In my own life, I always say, "Mama plans, baby laughs"! We never know quite where our children will take us, but if we follow and respond to their cues, the results are usually remarkable!

Tandem Nursing can be a remarkable journey. For many of us who have had the awe-inspiring privilege of nurturing two siblings at our breasts, it has been an extraordinary experience. There is nothing quite like the Peace of two small beings nestled together, drinking or dozing in quiet companionship.

Sometimes there may be small elbows digging into even smaller cheeks, and toes poking noses, but the memory of a dozen of these raucous moments is quickly erased by the timeless sight of two small hands quietly clasped amidst the rhythmic sounds of gulping, followed by the satiated slumber of completely relaxed children. The tenderness of an elder brother or sister towards a younger, sharing in the overflowing bounty of nourishment, is a precious reward, and safe harbor (if often a transient one) amid the daily tumult that is life with young children.

I hope that many more families will continue to find the information and support that they need to consider this remarkable path to meeting the needs of multiple children.

APPENDIX – RESOURCES

Finding Support

Many breastfeeding journeys would be smoother with more support. You, your baby, and your whole family deserve all you can get! It can be helpful to learn about the resources available in your area before you are in the thick of things and need help right away.

A great way to start is by finding your local "Peer Support Group" and attending an in-person meeting to get to know other nursing families, as well as trained Peer Support Counselors who can help with many common breastfeeding challenges. La Leche League is a great resource with free peer support for nursing families. It is a nonprofit organization staffed primarily by trained volunteers. La Leche League was founded in the United States, and now has both face-to-face and online meetings in over 60 countries around the world.

Other organizations are more country-specific, such as Breastfeeding USA in the United States, and the Australian Breastfeeding Association in Australia. All have websites where you can locate your nearest local group.

If you use Facebook, there are several discussion groups specifically for tandem nursing families. La Leche League has its own online Facebook discussion group about tandem nursing where families can both learn from each other's experiences, and hear from trained La Leche League Leaders providing evidence based information, at www.facebook.com/groups/llltandemnursing/

If you are a reader, keep your eyes out for the latest revised edition of *Adventures in Tandem Nursing*, by Hilary Flower. This is the most detailed and comprehensive written resource available on tandem nursing. Unfortunately as of this writing it is out of print and difficult to find, but a new edition is planned soon. In the meantime you may be able to find it through a public library, or a local La Leche League Group Library.

If you find you need more clinical support that goes beyond "normal course of breastfeeding" challenges, you should seek out an International Board Certified Lactation Consultant (IBCLC). You can find a listing of IBCLCs on the website of their professional association, the International Lactation Consultants Association (ILCA), at www.ilca.org. You may want to ask IBCLCs that you speak with whether they are familiar with tandem nursing so that you can find one who is attuned to your situation. Your IBCLC can work collaboratively with any doctors who are caring for you and your baby as a part of your healthcare team.

Working With Your Doctor

Working with physicians who are unfamiliar with tandem nursing, or even with the intricacies of nursing a single child, can be an added challenge when seeking breastfeeding support. Most physicians, whether obstetricians or pediatricians, receive little or no training in breastfeeding support during their medical education. Consequently they may offer information related to breastfeeding that is based on personal opinion, their own parenting philosophy, or cultural biases, rather than on medical training or research. Sharing evidence based information sources with your doctors can help to ease the way for the next patients and allow you to work collaboratively with your physician.

Some great information to share with your doctor about breastfeeding can be found online from the Academy of Breastfeeding Medicine. Their protocols are carefully researched documents written by *and for* physicians. The American Academy of Family Physicians *Statement on Nursing Beyond Infancy* can also be helpful to share with doctors unfamiliar with nursing during pregnancy and beyond. And with specific questions you can reach out to your local Peer Support Counselor to ask for evidence based sources to share and discuss with your doctor.

ABOUT THE AUTHOR

Sarah Shapiro is an IBCLC (Internationally Board Certified Lactation Consultant) and an active La Leche League Leader (a Peer Support Breastfeeding Counselor).

She has managed commercial vegetable farms and worked in farmland conservation in addition to breastfeeding and raising her own children. Supporting people and communities and helping them to thrive has always been a passion of hers.

Sarah lives in New York's Hudson Valley with her husband and children.

Printed in Great Britain
by Amazon